Letters To A Sex Addict

The Journey through Grief and Betrayal

Wendy Conquest

ISBN: 148956244-3
ISBN 13: 9781489562449
Library of Congress Control Number: 2013910108
CreateSpace Independent Publishing Platform
North Charleston, South Carolina

Praise for
Letters to a Sex Addict

"What does it feel like to be sexually betrayed? How does one cope and move on towards healing? This powerful collection of emotional letters written from the perspective of partners of sex addicts answers these questions and more. This simple book reveals the complex challenges of loving someone whose out-of-control sexual behavior has cracked the very foundations of love, trust, and intimacy in a committed relationship."

- Wendy Maltz, LCSW, DST, coauthor of *The Porn Trap: The Essential Guide to Overcoming Problems Caused by Pornography*

"In *Letters To A Sex Addict*, Wendy Conquest creatively brings together the soulful voices of partners of sex addicts. At a time when new technologies are altering sexual arousal patterns and stretching what is regarded as acceptable sexual behavior, this collection of eloquent and profound letters reminds us that sexual addiction violates trust and painfully impacts others. This book is sure to find its way into the hands of all those concerned with the consequences of sexual betrayal.

- Kenneth M. Adams, Ph.D., CSAT-S, author of *Silently Seduced* and *When He's Married to Mom*

"Wendy Conquest boldly captures the raw pain and emotion that partners experience when they discover they've been betrayed. The rich letters provide comfort and support to the betrayed partner by letting them know they are not alone. Others have been in that same dark place and have emerged into the arms of hope and healing. Therapists will certainly want to use this incredible resource in their practice with partners, sex addicts and couples."

-Stefanie Carnes, PhD, LMFT, author of *Mending A Shattered Heart* and *Facing Heartbreak*

To all those suffering.....

Foreword

BY ROBERT WEISS LCSW, CSAT-S

In her moving compilation, "Letters to a Sex Addict" therapist and clinical leader Wendy Conquest has beautifully illustrated the painful losses and harm experienced by those spouses who have sadly learned about their partner's ongoing pattern of betrayal. As Wendy so poignantly describes in this book, it's not so much the extramarital sex itself or any specific affair that causes spouses the deepest pain; instead, what hurts committed partners the most is the loss of their very ability to trust the person closest to them. Betrayal shatters trust. And it can be very, very difficult to reassemble the pieces of these kinds of broken relationships. The many personal and intimate "letters" Wendy has created here perfectly exemplify these points.

The simple truth is that for a healthy, attached primary partner to suddenly learn that they have been victimized by a profound emotional and/or sexual betrayal is incredibly traumatic. In fact, one study of women who unexpectedly learned of their husband's sexual addiction (and the related patterns of infidelity) found that a typical outcome of this kind of experience is a series of acute stress symptoms, very similar to the characteristics seen in post-traumatic stress disorder – which is a very legitimate and serious psychological condition.

Sadly, it is only over the past decade or so that the aftermath of intimate betrayal has become a legitimate area of study. As such, many family counselors and psychotherapists are behind the times in terms of helping betrayed individuals to identify and move past the traumatic, long-term effects of emotional and sexual betrayal. The good news is that psychotherapists and family counselors are slowly but steadily becoming more aware of- and open to- spotting the oftentimes fragile, rollercoaster-like, hyper-vigilant emotional state of the betrayed spouse. Typically, the trauma evoked by profound relationship betrayal manifests in one or more of the following ways:

- Emotional instability – quick shifts from rage to sadness to hope and back again

- Hyper-vigilance – endless questioning and secretive "detective work" (checking bills, wallets, browser histories, phone apps, and the like)

- Obsessing about the trauma – struggling to focus on day-to-day life, being easily distracted, etc.

- Depression – isolating, trouble sleeping or waking up, loss of interest in previously enjoyable activities, etc.

- Compulsive behaviors – drinking, drugging, shopping, gambling, and the like, in an effort to dull the pain

- Boundary problems like telling young children what dad or mom did. Telling bosses, family etc.

- Blaming themselves as the sole cause of the straying, the lying and the acting out

- Denial – avoiding thinking about or discussing the betrayal, and acting as if it didn't happen

- Trying to "reverse" the past- by having more sex with the betrayer, trying to lose weight, having plastic surgery, trying to become more alluring, etc.

All of the above reactions are seen repeatedly throughout this book. This issue alone makes this book helpful to readers, as betrayed spouses can often feel like the thoughts and emotions racing through their minds are unique to them. Learning by reading these pages that they are not alone is a comfort, offering the kind of light that can guide them toward the necessary healthy next steps required to get on with their lives.

In part, the trauma of infidelity stems from the fact that while the betraying individual or sex addict has obviously known about his or her sexual acting out all along and may actually be feeling some relief once the truth is revealed, betrayed spouses are typically blindsided by the information. And even in cases where the betrayed spouse was not fully in the dark, having some prior knowledge of the cheating, he or she is often overwhelmed by the full extent of the behavior – because, let's face it, a sex addict's infidelity is nearly always part of an ongoing pattern rather than an isolated incident. And it doesn't matter if that infidelity occurs online, out of town or in-person. As the letters in this book reveal, a sex addicts patterns of compulsive masturbation, often while viewing porn hour after hour, can feel just as devastating to a beloved spouse as does a "live" affair with a neighbor or coworker.

Making matters worse is the fact that betrayed spouses have sometimes had their "reality" denied for years by the cheating partner, who (most often attempting to cover up and protect their secret life), insists that he or she is not cheating, really did need to work until midnight, is not behaving differently, is not distant, and worse, that the worried spouse is being paranoid, mistrustful, and unfair.

Is it any wonder that when the cheated-on spouses of sex addicts finally find out they were right all along that they sometimes look like the crazy one?

The simple truth is this: As survivors of deep relationship trauma it is perfectly natural for spouses of sex addicts to respond with rage, tearfulness, or any other emotion when later 'triggered' by something seemingly as innocuous as the cheating spouse coming home from work five minutes later than expected. Until relationship trust is re-established, which can take a year or longer, betrayed spouses are likely to spin-cycle through anger, fear, distrust, confusion, and then repeat. And these reactions are perfectly normal and not to be pathologized.

Sadly, partners of sex addicts are usually angry not only with their cheating spouse, but with themselves. Some have already turned to alcohol abuse, drugs, overeating, compulsive spending, gambling, and the like as a way to self-soothe and numb the pain of living with a non-intimate, unavailable, and dishonest partner. Others may "cheat back" as a form of retaliation, only to later hate themselves for doing it. Still others simply beat themselves up emotionally for not seeing the infidelity that was seemingly so obvious to everyone else. None of these reactions are right or wrong; they just are, and we see them illustrated with care and thoughtful reflection throughout this fine book.

I am particularly pleased that Wendy has chosen not to present a Pollyanna ending to the book. Yes, some (actually most) partners of sex addicts choose to remain in their relationships – reestablishing trust and comfort with their sex addicted spouse over a period of many months or even years. However, for some cheated-on spouses the pain of betrayal is simply too much, and the violation they have experienced is greater than their desire to remain in the marriage. For these men and women trust cannot be restored – Humpty Dumpty cannot be glued back together again. In such cases, ending the marriage may well be the best solution. In the end, what is most important for betrayed spouses to find is a healthy way to grieve and grow beyond their loss. This always means placing a renewed emphasis on trusting their own instincts, a greater willingness to trust and express their emotions (including fear), while establishing and maintaining a support network of both peers and professionals.

It is my hope that this highly evocative text will offer those suffering from the painful loss of betrayal an understanding that they are not alone, that other smart, engaged and caring partners have also been unknowingly been betrayed. And importantly, that the wild array of feelings they are likely experiencing and everything in between, can be a quite healthy response for anyone whose sense has been deeply shaken. These men and women need to know, as Ms. Conquest has gently reminded them, that they do not have to move forward alone – even if they decide to walk away from their relationship.

Robert Weiss LCSW, CSAT-S is Senior Vice President of Clinical Development with Elements Behavioral Health. A licensed UCLA MSW graduate and personal trainee of Dr. Patrick Carnes, he founded The Sexual Recovery Institute in Los Angeles in 1995. He is author of Cruise Control: Understanding Sex Addiction in Gay Men, and co-author with Dr. Jennifer Schneider of both Untangling the Web: Sex, Porn, and Fantasy Obsession in the Internet Age and his newest release, Closer Together, Further Apart: The Effect of Technology and the Internet on Sex, Intimacy and Relationships, along with numerous peer-reviewed articles and chapters.

TABLE OF CONTENTS

Introduction

Welcome to *Letters to a Sex Addict*. This book's purpose is to help you understand the experience of being the partner of someone who is sexually compulsive. You will discover many different aspects of the internal workings that happen when a husband or wife has found out there have been lies and betrayal within a committed relationship. If you are a partner, I suggest you read this book however you see fit. You may want to look at the table of contents and pick a topic that seems to be happening at the moment. You may want to start at the beginning of the book and read through to the end.

This book was constructed to help mitigate the challenges of reading when trauma is present. It was written with the expectation that the reader would be going back to it throughout her or his experience. That being said, healing from this situation takes time. Every person I have worked with has been anxious to get over the pain as quickly as possible, and to have his or her partner further along in recovery.

This is a journey, and you will be changed by it forever. However, the destruction does not have to eat away at your soul. You can heal and transform this poison into something that makes you stronger, wiser, more sensitive and courageous.

If you are a sex addict, or think you may have a problem with sex, these letters will reveal what your partner is thinking and feeling in a very direct way. If you feel ashamed, angry, indignant or depressed, I suggest you see a therapist who is certified in sex addiction, and begin attending 12-step "S" groups; SAA, SLAA, and/or SA. These meetings provide support, understanding, compassion and a program to stop your behaviors and live a more meaningful life. If you have just been "discovered" NOW is the time to get help. You will not be able to control or stop these behaviors on your own if you are an addict. There are resources listed in the Where To Go For Help section.

When I first began working with partners of sex addicts, I wondered if there would be a difference between someone whose partner "only" watched pornography and those whose significant others were actually having sex with other people. What I found repeatedly is *there is no difference.* Lying, taking attention away from the relationship, and creating feelings of rejection register the same in the partner.

We are learning more daily about porn and sex addiction; how they are similar and how they differ. The majority of sex addicts started viewing porn before their behaviors escalated. Our culture has accepted pornography as being part of our collective sexuality. In general, whether heterosexual, gay, lesbian, trans-gendered, married, engaged, or single, my clients report pornography erodes the relationship over time rather than enhancing intimacy.

We are wired to attach to other human beings. We are hurt when we lie and when we are lied to. When we are chronically betrayed, our reality, self-esteem, healthy sense of sexuality, trust, and safety are severely impacted.

The letters are a compilation of experiences from clients, friends, family and my own history. If you hear yourself in one of them, it is because you are not alone. You will not relate to all of the words. Take what is relevant for you. In addition, if you read this book at different times over your process, your resonance with different letters may change.

From my heart to yours, I hope this book helps in your process of understanding yourself and your partner.

* The content herein is not any individual's life story but a composite from hundreds of clients the author has treated.

Defining Sexual Addiction

This book's title is *Letters to a Sex Addict,* and so I feel it is important to talk about what sex addiction is. The widely accepted definition of addiction is anything that evolves in a behavior beyond a person's control. There are two major categories now; one is chemical, which would include alcohol, cocaine, painkillers, marijuana, and other drugs, and the other is behavioral. Behavioral addictions include shopping, eating, gambling, on-line gaming, and sex. My belief is that behavioral addictions are more challenging to arrest than chemical addictions. A person can walk out of a bar but we can't stop eating.

The two main factors defining sex addiction are the same as with all other addictions: an inability to stop despite repeated efforts to do so, and, an escalation with frequency and increased risk-taking. For addiction to be treated effectively, the person needs to be motivated and willing to admit that their behavior has become uncontrollable and unmanageable AND that they need help. Most individuals seek professional therapy from a therapist that specializes in the particular compulsivity they are struggling with, i.e., a person struggling with pornography addiction would seek out a Certified Sex Addiction Therapist. There are few who can overcome any addiction without a community who understands and people who can hold that person accountable.

PART ONE:

In the Dark

To be trusted is a greater compliment than being loved.

- George MacDonald

Life, before we realize betrayal, can have many varying aspects to it. Some partners will say they really had no knowledge of anything wrong. Others will say they suspected something but couldn't quite put their finger on it. Partners have been subjected to being blamed of being in denial; that they really *did* know something was amiss, but couldn't face the truth or confront their husband because of their own fear or co-dependency. What I know is that sexual betrayal by someone you are attached to is likened to hearing wolves howling at the window....you aren't going to open the door.

Derailed – Columbia, South Carolina

I'm sensing a change in our relationship that I don't understand, and it has me on edge. It's not anything specific, but something has definitely changed. When I came to the office to bring some food for your staff, no one would look at me. I could feel the tension in the air. What's that about? These people were always so friendly and open with me, and now they won't even look at me.

You "uninvited" me to the company Christmas party at the last minute, but you're still going. Why are spouses not invited all of a sudden? And why are you working so late these last few weeks? You've never had to stay so late before.

You used to want me to come to bed whenever you were ready for the night, but lately you're going to bed alone, without asking me if I'm tired. And when I come to bed, you're already asleep.

All in Your Head – Los Angeles, California

Mindy, are you cheating on me? I went over to your house and there was a man's t-shirt there on the couch. You told me the guys on your text messages were just friends. You tell me the guys on your Facebook page are people you don't know that well. I just can't believe it.

The other day I was checking the phone bill and there was one number with hours of time. When I asked if I could see your phone, you said "no." When I confronted you with the phone calls, you said it was your new boss's number. Now that made me mad. When I asked what his name is, you said it was none of my business. How the hell can I believe you? This is making me crazy.

Left Out – Boulder, Colorado

I don't think I have ever written you a letter. I've given you notes in cards but I don't remember an actual letter. Well, I guess the time has come.

There are a lot of things on my mind and a lot of sorrow in my heart. Things have come to the surface for me tonight. After working for your company all day, not being able to reach you by phone or text, and coming home to an empty house, I feel so used and disrespected and unimportant. More than that, I feel unloved and unappreciated.

Reaching Out – Chicago. Illinois

I wanted to write to you. I've been thinking of
all the amazing ways you have helped me in my
life and I wanted to share that with you.

Without you I don't think I would have ever "grown up." To
begin, you taught me how to have a career. (Remember you
saying that you have to have a career in order to retire? I'll never
forget that. I was so mad, but you were so right!) All the twists
and turns in my becoming able to have my own company and
you were right there with each choice, and each letting go.

You have always supported me in everything that I wanted to
do. Even when I quit my full-time job, remember? I think you
said, "I didn't think you'd actually do it!" You're the best!

Texts – Dallas, Texas

Hey! I need to ask you about this really weird text message I saw on your phone. It said something about "this is Fire and Ice, we're ready when you are." I know you have said that these sorts of texts accidentally come on your phone from time to time, but I don't understand how that happens.

Also, you've been really moody and I don't know how to help. Is there anything I can do? I love you and our life together so much. How about if I make your favorite dinner this weekend? Then maybe we can go for a walk? I would like that.

Ok, I hope you are having a great day!

Again – Myrtle Beach, South Carolina

Is it happening again? I thought we were over this. I
really believed that we had a new start when we left
the northeast and all the bad memories there. Your
"indiscretions" were behind us. The whispers of ex-friends
were far away now and couldn't hurt us anymore.

I never believed what they said about you, about that girl you
took in your truck for a day. You were just giving her a new
experience. I didn't believe that the secretary in your company's
office was crushing on you. Well, maybe she was, but you didn't
do anything about it. I know that in my heart. That "mistake"
you made, taking a prostitute in your truck one night, was an
aberration, something that will never happen again. When you
went on that cruise by yourself, and the women from the cruise
started to call and write you, I believed it was just because
you were so attentive. After all, they were all married, too.

But today, you were telling me that you treated yourself to a
two-hour lunch, and when I asked you who the lucky person
was who got to share that lunch, you didn't answer for a very
long moment. And then you said her name – the accountant
that everyone at your work always talks about. The one they
say is a man-eater and hones in on everyone's husband.

Is she honing in on you? And are you letting her?

I'm so uneasy. Something is wrong. Why won't you talk to me
about it? Just two months ago, we had a wonderful getaway at the
beach and we seemed on-track. Now I feel as if we're derailed.

Talk to me. Please.

Another Woman? – Baton Rouge, Louisiana

Here is what me and my girls
were talking about today:

"You know, Sholanda, I think
he may be cheatin'."

"What you talking 'bout? You got
one o' the good ones!"

"Yeah, I'm not so sure 'bout that."

So I'm askin' – Is you or is
you not fuckin' around?

PART TWO:
Discovery

Three things cannot be long hidden: the sun, the moon, and the truth.

- Buddha

When we first know, with certainty, that our loved one has strayed, it is a moment that will define everything that comes after it. People in the sex addiction field call this time, "Discovery." Our minds and bodies work together to identify and create safety. When we realize we have been lied to, our whole world tips on its axis as we lose the balance of our everyday lives. We often react in strange and unexpected ways, similar to the way we would react to a natural disaster. I like to explain this experience as holding a puzzle board that had all the aspects of your life beautifully connected, suddenly being thrown up into the air, and you are now staring at a blank slate surrounded by hundreds of confusing, unconnected pieces.

Crisis! – San Francisco, California

I cannot calm down. I feel adrenaline coursing through my body all the time. Every nerve in my body is tingling and my stomach is in knots. This feeling is familiar to me. It reminds me when I'd come home as a kid and my dad would be waiting, angry. This reminds me of when I first went off to school and I was all on my own for the very first time. My therapist says I need to tell the difference between excitement and fear and anxiety. I have no idea what she is talking about.

What I do know is that I can't be in this state forever. I want to believe that I can handle this and it will fade, but secretly, I know this will hurt me if it continues.

I think a piece of me has gone crazy. I don't want to say that too loud. I don't want to admit how this has affected me. The cat puked on the floor yesterday and I came unglued! My low fuel warning beeped while I was driving and I thought I was running out of gas at that minute. It's as if the part of me that knows I'll be okay has disappeared. And so everything is a crisis these days. I panic at the slightest things and am in a constant state of anxiety. I don't like this. I can't live like this.

I Don't Understand – Lincoln, Nebraska

You've hurt me. I know this is hard to hear. But
this pain drops down so deep. You were the one I
wanted to be with. You were the one I trusted with
my personal fears, joys, hopes and dreams. They
say that you have a disease; that this is some sort
of brain malfunctioning. To me it sounds like an
excuse. I'm hurt and angry. I don't understand how
you could do this to me. I don't understand how you
could do this to our family. I don't understand how
you could do this to our church and to God. I want
to swear at you, hit you, kick you, and make you
realize how this has affected me because you don't
get it! And when you dare accuse me that somehow
this is my fault, I am beside myself with rage.

You lied to me.

You preferred other women to me.

You made me believe you loved me.

You took what was sacred and made it a mockery.

You were selfish.

You were mean.

You betrayed our entire life together.

How Did I Get Here? - San Antonio, Texas

I can't eat. I can't sleep. And I throw up. My mind and my body are in a state of fear and shock. I find myself doing ridiculous things like hiding what I think are important things like my passport, or money, or an extra set of keys. I have no idea what my future holds and I am thinking crazy, irrational thoughts.

Depending on what you have told me, I am thinking of calling your boss, or the woman you are having the affair with, or her husband. I may want to tell everyone what an asshole you are; or I may want to keep this terrible secret to myself.

Regardless, I feel very scared and hurt and alone. I don't know what to do, what to say, or where to go.

I'm told this may last weeks or months; this process could even last for years. I guess it really depends on many things; one being your attitude, another being your actions, yet another being how well I can ask for help, and how well I can set boundaries. What has happened and how did we get here???

Denial – Bozeman, Montana

I know you've done horrible things and I don't want to know. I'm really scared. I'm scared for me, for our family, for our children. The first thing I have to be assured of is that our children are safe. If they are in harm's way, I need to leave.

When the wolves are outside, you aren't going to open the door. You aren't going to peek through the window either. There has been howling for a long time and I haven't dared to think of the danger that lurks just on the other side of the wall. So I've pretended I don't hear it. I've wrapped myself up in the pretty memories of us and our family. This has been my life preserver as I have persevered as a wife and a mother. I know now some of what you have done. I still am having a very difficult time imagining who and what else has happened. A big part of me needs to know, and a bigger part of me insists on not knowing. Because once I know, what can I do with that? How can I possibly handle knowing the whole truth about you?

My Truth – New York City, New York

You're Sick.

Only Me – San Francisco, California

I thought you thought I was pretty and sexy and attractive.
You would tell me I was. But there were those times where
you would pull away and I would wonder. I convinced myself
that you were over-worked or stressed by the children or
by your family. Sometimes I would wonder if you might be
having an affair. And when I asked you if this was possible
you would either reassure me that you weren't, or you would
brush me off as being silly or crazy. But I wasn't either of those
things. A part of me knew something was wrong, but I didn't
have enough proof. There was no "one thing" I could point
to and say, "That's it! That's what's wrong." And how could
I tell the kids I was leaving on just a feeling or a hunch?

Now I want you to tell me that you want me and only
me. When I ask you to say you thought that other
woman was ugly, or stupid, or a whore, it's because I
want to know you DON'T want to be with HER.

And sometimes you look at me and try to explain how she was
attractive in her own way. Or you defend her somehow. And
at these times I feel so much! I feel like killing you; I feel like
killing myself. Or I feel like just disappearing. I try to get you to
understand how wrong this all was. And then I feel like giving up.

Know when I demand that you trash her very *existence*,
it is because I am fighting for my place as your wife,
your partner, the mother of your children.

Oblivious – Fort Collins, Colorado

I feel I have given you *everything* and our
children *everything*. Some say I have given
too much, but this is how I was raised;
to give is to love. Now that there are
times when I have asked you to leave, I
experience many different feelings. One
feeling, honestly, is relief. I thought I
would feel very sad, but that is not the
case. I still am trying to figure things
out; to get a better understanding why this
happened and why it happened now. Why not
earlier in our relationship, or later?

I think you know what I have given to you
and our family. I wonder if you know and
appreciate all of it though. I feel I have
had to overcompensate with parenting. You
just aren't fully there for our children. I
feel I have had to work harder at figuring
out our finances; you have fought me with
having a budget for years. I have taken
care of re-modeling jobs, moving when we
sold our home, preparing or providing meals
for our whole family. I've made sure there

were birthday presents, Christmas presents, presents for our kids' birthday parties; presents for our friends' house warming parties. I've made sure your mom and dad came over for dinner for their anniversary. I made sure the animals were fed, bathed and taken to the vet. The list goes on and on. Do you see everything I have contributed? Do you care? From making sure the house is clean to swapping out old toothbrushes, I get the feeling you think these things just happen!

Blame – Rochester, NY

Now you're blaming me for your sexual behavior. You're saying I just didn't do it for you anymore, that you weren't attracted to me in the way you used to be. Maybe you are saying I'm not sexy enough, or don't give you enough sex. Maybe you are saying I just don't understand you.

Hmmm. It's true. I have settled into marriage. I have settled into being with just you. We have dogs together, kids together, a house together. I have seen the stray hair on your back day after day. I have heard you pass gas when you thought no one was there to hear. I have seen your body changing in not so attractive ways. I have been there for you when work wasn't going well. I have been there for you when there were problems with your family. I was there for you, loving you when you were at your worst.

And now you say I don't do it for you. I want to take those words and stuff them down your throat. I want everyone you love to leave you. I want to cut your head off with a saber and watch you bleed to death. I want you to grow old and be alone. This is the rage I feel, like Pele bursting and destroying everything. Pele spews fire and lava to create new land. I can't see a new beginning now. If you come to me and want me to forgive you, it will be a long, long time and then only after I heal from these gaping wounds. You will never know, really, the pain you have caused.

Being Honest – Phoenix, Arizona

Now that we both know what you have been
doing, you want to tell me the whole truth.
You now want to be "honest." You are sharing
information about who you were with, what you
did, what you liked and didn't like sexually, maybe
relationally. You are filling my head with pictures
and details that I think I want to know, but I really
don't. I am trying to put together what the hell
happened to you, to me, to our relationship.

What I need is for you to be working with a
professional who will help you categorize and figure
out the progression of your behaviors. I also really
need you to try and figure out why this happened.
I understand you feel bad about what happened. I
get that you are trying to put the pieces together
yourself. But when you say how good the sex was
with another woman, this makes me feel like crap.
Or how you really tried not to look at porn, but just
couldn't stop. If you plan on staying with me, and
you plan on us having a good sex life, ever, then
you will not give me information before both of us
are ready. This is not about being honest. This is
about you trying to relieve your guilt. Or trying to

figure out what this is all about. All you're doing now is making me feel bad. I feel devastated by what you've done, because whether you realize it or not, you've destroyed a piece of me.

Honesty for me is when you start telling me where you are going, what you are doing, and who you are with, without me having to ask.

Honesty is you sharing with me how your therapy sessions are going, or your 12 step meeting, without sharing what other people are doing, or how much better you are than them.

Honesty is not withholding information about anything, but being discerning.

Honesty is about sharing your internal world with me minus the whatever thoughts and compulsions you have that are part of your addict.

I Look Good on the Outside – Miami, Florida

I have always prided myself with keeping myself together and looking good. And I am still doing that today. I don't want many people to know the pain I am in unless they can directly relate to what I am going through. And I believe no one really gets it.

I think it is strange when friends come over and we pretend that everything is ok. I feel like a ghost wandering around my own house. I'm here, making the same meals, entertaining the same people, picking up the same clothes, but I'm just going through the motions. You may think when you see me that everything is fine. And you have always known me to be strong, so you may think I am through the worst of this ordeal. I'm not. When I'm alone, I cry. When I'm with friends, I feel isolated or crazy. When I'm with the kids, I am stuffing my feelings down because I don't want to expose them to this poison I feel inside.

I'm doing the best I can, and I feel the need to stay busy. The worst thing I can do is assume all is well. I cannot ignore my own needs and continue to take responsibility for what you have done. I am holding myself together. Somewhere along the line I learned this is what I had to do. Maybe it was when I was a child or a teenager. Maybe I learned to be this independent as a young adult. This is a quality I think you have liked about me. Maybe you even counted on it. But know it feels like a brittle shell about to break. I'm afraid if it does crack and crumble, I will evaporate into nothingness.

Irritability – Newport, Rhode Island

I've been irritable. This feeling is as if someone had stuck a very thin sliver of wood under my tailbone. It's always there, difficult to reach and perhaps I am not even sure what it is - only that I want it to go away. Even though my mood and behavior declare differently, I pretend nothing is wrong. I think about that presentation scheduled for Wednesday at work and a snarling dragon emerges up my spine and into my jaw. I actually hear myself snort. I don't want to do it. My chest starts to tense and I think of who I can blame for getting me into this situation.

Then I go back to brandishing my sword to root out who trapped me into this dismal situation. I think it was my mother. It's HER fault, somehow. Maybe it's my dad's shortcoming. He was never able to follow through with anything! He'd start working on the classic car he was re-building and half way through he'd leave it in pieces to go get a beer, or a whiskey. Despite my mother's begging for him to finish, it remained a pile of rubbish instead of the intended restored beauty.

I try to strategize how to remove this feeling, like a surgeon without the proper tools. Watch TV? Go for a run. Maybe I should eat something; maybe I'm hungry. No, I'm just angry. I'm overwhelmed and realize the house is a mess, I need to call the bank, I said I'd meet with my manager, the post office closes at five, and I have to get a haircut. My heart starts to race and my breathing gets shallow and now that sliver of wood has become an electric current racing through my body. Irritation leads to panic and now my mind is racing and my body is reacting. I feel like I am going to throw up, or bang my head against the wall, or worse.

The phone rings. As I answer my mind snaps to a different place. By the end of the conversation I do not know what place I will be in; distracted or calmed or back in the fire. This is my life. This is my hell.

Staying; Leaving – Salt Lake City, Utah

Should I stay or should I leave? If I leave how do I explain a divorce to my children? They shouldn't know about your sexual immoral behavior. And I don't even know how to explain that to them. They should know. They should know how you have hurt me! No, I can't hurt them like that. Telling would only confuse them.

Maybe they have seen you on the computer. Have they seen you watching porn? Have they seen you masturbating? You covered up and lied to me, so maybe they have caught you, walked in on you....I need to leave you. I love you so much!

I feel this zinging throughout my body. My heart is racing. Adrenaline is surging. My head is spinning, and I can't quite catch my breath. I find myself sighing...a lot. I should leave, I can't leave, I hate you, I love you, how could you do this to me; to us? Could you pick up some bacon and eggs on your way home?

Razor's Edge – Los Angeles, California

Qquueeek, qqquuueeeek, qqqquuueeeeekkkkkkk. Like a wind-up ballerina in a jewelry box the metal coil inside of me gets tighter and tighter. My stomach feels cramped and irritated; my head is trapped in a vice, which allows my neck no movement at all. *Pretty, must look pretty*, float the words in my brain. They swirl like some trapeze artist high in the ethers of a circus tent. I go to work, but am in a daze. I feel I can't move in any direction. I think I have to keep a smile on my face for friends, family, our children, my co-workers. I'm exhausted with trying to find sanity and so I just collapse when I am by myself. The people I have shared with are tired of hearing about my problems, and I feel there is no one who really understands.

Knowing that you had two lives has created the same for me, ironically. How I am staying focused with work, or with the kids, I can't explain. I just know I have to keep myself from falling apart. I have been told I am controlling in the past. Now I challenge anyone to cross me as I try to keep some semblance of a life together. Controlling. Perhaps I wasn't controlling enough. Maybe if I had been more demanding and managing this wouldn't have happened!

A tiny voice inside of me says that if I don't do something different I'm going to be in severe trouble. But I don't know what to do. Therapists I go to either look at me with pity, or shock and confusion. How can they help me if they can't understand? I feel like I'm on a razor's edge between sanity and chaos.

Rage - Oklahoma City, Oklahoma

I have this almost uncontrollable impulse
to kill you. I'm shocked that I would say
this let alone that I feel this way. I don't
know where it comes from and it scares me.
I have violent thoughts. I think of taking
the computer where you were watching porn
and slamming it into your face. I think
about burning the car you had sex in,
sometimes with you in it. I want to hit,
strangle, stab you; rip your clothes, bite
and scratch and punch the shit out of you.

I was told I have herpes when I went to the
doctor's office. The doctor isn't sure you
gave it to me, but I am. I've never had an
STD before so this is another thing you've
given me. I'm waiting for the entire screen
of tests to come back. I'm half-hoping
there's more so I can hate you more......

I read somewhere that when animals are
severely threatened, to the point of death,
they rise up and attack their predator even
if the other animal is twenty times their

size. They go from a place of immobilization to moving to kill. It's the last chance they have for survival. I'm wondering if this is what I'm experiencing. This feeling is so primal and irrational. I guess I need you to know I don't know what this is, and I'm as scared as you are when it happens.

Porn – Las Vegas, Nevada

You've been looking at those women. I don't know if
they are older, thinner, or have bigger tits than me.
Every girl I know feels weird about her body, and it's the
same with me. Girls compare themselves to other girls
all the time. So now your job is to convince me that it
is my body you want, my ass you desire. This ain't
going to be an easy ride. Somehow you need to cough
up why those whores, who you jacked off to and ogled
for hours on end, are not in your frickin' head now.

Also you were watching porn with nasty stuff I don't like.
You need to figure this out too. In my mind I want to please
you, and at the same time I don't want to do stuff I'm not
comfortable with. I've been taught that certain things are
dirty, and now it feels like you like that dirty stuff. And
I'm not keen on my own stuff either. When I know you are
looking at this, I just hate myself and you at the same time.

Not my problem. – Minneapolis, Minnesota

I understand now that you are saying you have a sex addiction. And I don't understand why I am spending time reading books, going to support groups, going to therapy. This is your problem, not mine.

Why can't our life, my life, just be simple? When we were going to couples counseling you should have told that therapist what was going on with you. But you didn't. You had so many opportunities to stop. But you didn't. You decided not to. You didn't once consider what you were doing to me. So why should I now be a part of this whole mess? Can't you just go and get fixed? For me, for you, just fix it!

Shock – Knoxville, Tennessee

I don't think I realized what shock was before now. I would have said I did. And I've always been very good at crises. I've been good at fixing and managing. Some people would say I'm controlling. But this situation is different. I don't know what to say and I don't know how to react.

I'm pushing myself. I'm relying on old, old coping skills. I'm acting and reacting in ways I haven't since I was a girl. I hate myself for this. There are times when I feel strong and keep everything together, as I always have. If only I can control you, your behavior, our home, the children, my work and the dog, then, maybe this didn't happen, or maybe I can get through this.

And then I collapse. I feel I'm going crazy and I can't move. I do one of two things. I either get more controlling or I lose it in hysterics of how awful you are and how you've destroyed everything. I rant; I rave. I might hit you. I might throw things; break things. Nothing else matters anymore. And I think I just go numb.

I don't like being this way. And I can't seem to stop.

And the awful thing is …I don't know how this is going to go. Will I change in a week, a month, a year? I'm scared I will never be able to get beyond what happened. I'm scared I'll get hurt again. I'm scared we won't make it.

Why Me? - Boston, Massachusetts

I'm not a Buddhist, but I'm wondering about karma. What the hell did I do to deserve this? I try not to go to this place but I really am trying to figure out why this happened and why to me. I've tried really hard to be a good person. I've tried to do the right things in life. I don't understand why this has happened not just once but now multiple times. Are you just out to get me? Are you just trying to hurt me as much as you can? Why WHY stay married if this other life is what you want? Just go! Go live the life of a single woman! Why drag me down over and over again?

Looking Back – Seattle, Washington

We were both married to other people when we met. How did I fool myself into believing that somehow what we had was different? That it was more special or that we understood each other better than anybody else? Oh, if there had only been someone who could have told me. But no one knew. I made sure to keep you and what we were doing hidden. You convinced me I was the one. And I wanted to be with you. One affair I might be able to handle, to understand, but you are telling me there were men all through our marriage. How am I supposed to face my friends? My family? And most of all, myself?

Acceptance – Paducah, Kentucky

This is not the life I expected. I didn't go into this relationship thinking I would be betrayed. I did not stay in this relationship to be hurt, even though I knew something was wrong. I feel I have been there for you and now I need you to be there for me. I don't know what I am going to need. Sometimes I will ask you for more; sometimes I will ask you for less. I won't know until the moment arises and my request may not be rational. But I need you to honor my request, no matter how illogical or irrational it may seem to you.

You are not the person I thought you were, and you will see a side to me you may never have seen before. I say this not to threaten or punish you. I say this to ask for acceptance as I try to find myself and deal with this horror.

The Worst - Lansing, Michigan

When you told me you were a drug addict, I wished you were an alcoholic. When you told me you were a sex addict, I would have given anything for you to be a drug addict.

I get this is a disease. And I'm starting to understand this chemical thing that happens in your brain.

The piece I am having trouble with is how you did your addiction. Never would I have thought you would get involved with friends of ours, or our neighbors. Never would I have believed you would use our hard-earned money to have sex with other women. The fact you brought a woman into our house and into our bed feels like the lowest betrayal and the meanest thing you could do. Watching porn is bad enough, but you watched when you were supposed to be caring for our children. It's not that you went to strip bars, but that you borrowed from our line of credit to do it and then didn't tell me. It's not just that you had sex with other women, but that you were "too tired" to have sex with me. It's not that you were watching porn on your computer, but that you watched porn on MY computer.

In addition, it's the timing of when your acting out happened. Again I am hearing from the experts that at times of greater intimacy you freak out and need to create distance. Ok, but when I was pregnant? When my mother was dying? When our daughter was getting married? The times in our lives that should have been the happiest were the worst.

Nothing is the same – Iowa City, Iowa

Don't buy me my favorite flowers. They
aren't my favorites anymore.

Don't call me by my pet name because I wonder
if that is what you called her as well.

Don't look at me as I undress because I feel
embarrassed and self-conscious by your gaze.

Don't take me to any restaurant you have been to with her.

Don't assume my birthday, your birthday or
our anniversary is a day of celebration.

Don't assume we are going on a family vacation this year.

If you bought me something special, I
wonder if you bought that for her too.

Photos of us together make me laugh, but not with joy.

Don't pretend that we are the same. Nothing is the same.

Wilted – Oak Brook Terrace, Illinois

I find myself not caring about anything. A volcano has exploded and is now quiet and somehow I have survived, but I am exhausted. I see you're happier and healthier but I am wrung out. When I look back over the last months, I don't know where the time went. And I don't know how I got through it at all. I used to love to go shopping, and now I have no desire. I used to enjoy a good book, and I don't want to read. I feel like I have lost and gained weight repeatedly, and now I just don't care. My children are the only thing that seems to give me some joy.

What has happened to me? I feel older but not in a good, wise way but in a flat, dejected way. I find myself not caring about things. When you ask me what I want to do on Sunday or what we should have for dinner, I don't have an opinion. Sometimes I feel like I could simply sit on the couch and stare out the window for days. I think the plants are getting watered and the pets are being fed. Many times I need to double check to see if this is true. Who am I? And will I get through this?

Hope – Casper, Wyoming

I can't believe what people are telling me. I don't WANT to believe it. I know guys look at porn. I know sometimes people stray outside the marriage. This doesn't mean anything is really wrong!

You know, I'm thinking we can handle this by ourselves. I think if we get help from our pastor and from friends and family, we can beat this thing! I love you so much. We have children together. There is no way this could be that bad. It's going to be okay.

We'll be all right.

We have to be.

PART THREE:
Unraveling

Hear my prayer, O Lord, and give ear unto my cry; hold not thy peace at my tears: for I am a stranger with thee, and a sojourner, as all my fathers were.

Psalms 39:12

After some time has gone by, you begin to see how you have been holding everything together. Perhaps your husband or wife has entered treatment or counseling; perhaps they are starting to attend recovery meetings. This is now the time where you unconsciously let go and start to breathe again. But this is also the time where you start to feel all of your feelings. And there are so many feelings that it's almost impossible to sort them out. As you emerge from the shock of discovery, you may feel grief, anger, fear, pain – both physical and emotional, hate, and even love. There may also be a fight or flight component, wherein you alternate between wanting to run away and needing to stand and fight for your relationship with the person who has caused your pain.

Confusion - Austin, Texas

I'm not myself. I'm forgetting where I put things.
I can't remember what bills I've paid. I find that
sometimes I'm driving too fast or too slow, usually
too fast. I'm forgetting important events like our
granddaughter's birthday or critical meetings at work.
If I was older I'd think this was menopause. Everyone
is suggesting in polite ways that I'm depressed.

There are some good days where I feel very productive and
get a lot done, but I don't know when these days are going
to be. On the worst days, I feel stuck and unable to move.
Little things like cleaning the bathroom seem to be the
most important task -above shopping for dinner, doing
the taxes, or even helping the kids with homework. None
of this makes sense and I'm embarrassed. After what's
happened, my self-esteem has been hit hard enough without
feeling that now I'm stupid and incompetent as well.

Commitment – Taos, New Mexico

Now I'm wondering if we can be together or not.
Your childhood was awful; mine was good! You
didn't have an available mom; well, that's putting it
lightly. In my opinion she was not a loving mother.
We argue about this a lot, with you defending her
and me trying to make a point. Anyway, my family
was close; yours wasn't.
I truly believe that I know what commitment
is, and your actions are showing that you
do not. How are you going to learn how to
just be with me? How are you going to know
what life you want? How are you going to
make up for all the harm you have done?

I wish if you hadn't wanted to get married, you
would have stood up and said that's not what
you wanted. You say over and over that you
wanted to be with me but you were scared. What
were you so afraid of? Was it that I wouldn't be
enough for you? That you couldn't be satisfied
with just one woman in your life? Did you
know back then that you had this problem?

You've also said I'm the only one you loved. Hard to believe when you left my birthday party to text another woman! Where was your commitment then? How can we both believe you can do this?

Consoling Me – Milwaukee, Wisconsin

I get that you want to make me feel better and maybe take away the pain. The WORST thing you can do is say you understand what I am feeling. Let me say this again another way. DO NOT TELL ME YOU UNDERSTAND HOW I FEEL. This is insulting, degrading, and invalidating.

Have you been in any relationship where you were lied to for the amount of time you lied to me? Did the other person watch porn as much as you did? Did your ex have sex with as many people as you have? Have you ever been with someone that made you believe nothing was wrong when <u>everything</u> was wrong? Have you worked your ass off taking care of family and work and finances and children while your partner was masturbating to porn or spending money in strip clubs or having sex with prostitutes? THEN, and only then, can you tell me you understand how I feel.

Please, if you want to console me, listen to what I need. I may not be the best at telling you and it may change from moment to moment. But thinking you have walked in my shoes is just plain wrong.

Two Lives – Augusta, Maine

I'm learning that I never really knew you. I thought we shared a life but you were somewhere else. I am learning that you have a certain look in your eyes that signals your mind is elsewhere. I am realizing that when you say mean things to me, that is your other side. I'm learning to ask direct questions, which I already know the answer to. I'm learning to be a detective, a police officer, and a prison marshal. I don't want to be any of these. I'm angry you have put this on me; on us. Why can't someone else be patrolling your computer? Why can't someone else be responsible for you when you travel?

Looking back I see the split we had. I'm realizing your dark side was there before we met. And I'm wondering how I was attracted to someone who wasn't fully there for me. Was I like a teenage girl who thinks they will change the "bad boy" of the school if she just loves him enough? Or did I like the distance because then there weren't too many demands on me?

I'm wondering if we can heal this. Some people say this sex addiction thing brought them closer together. That's hard for me to imagine since I thought we were close in a lot of ways. My family was not that close. We were there for each other; more so than your family, but I wonder if I know what real emotional intimacy is.

We've been this way for so long I don't know how to change. I know you have to stop your acting out. I can't have another betrayal. The reading I'm doing says you can't do it alone. You aren't a person who likes asking for help. I don't know how you're going to succeed. It's not that I don't believe in you I just think it will take a lot to do something different.

I wonder if you want a life together with me. Or would you rather have a life with another? You may need to tell me many times that you want to be with me. You may need to tell me how your addiction works because it doesn't make sense to me. My mind can understand some of it some of the time, but my heart just hurts.

Sensitivity – Bloomington, Indiana

I have become hypersensitive. I've felt I was an intuitive person, but now I can't distinguish between the trauma and my right awareness. I walk into the room where the computer is and I freeze. There are days I can't even think of going in that room. I see women, normal women, with their pretty engagement rings and their shiny wedding bands, and I want to ask them if they know what their husband is doing right now. They THINK they know, but do they really?

I'll be watching my television program and an ad for women's underwear will come on. I can't bear to watch it, and I end up leaving the room to go and cry. You will say certain words or mention places that I can't bear to hear anymore. I'm sensitive to your drinking alcohol now because when you drank you would watch porn or be on the computer. When you are too quiet, I am hyper alert. Why are you quiet? What are you doing? Do I want to know?

Depression – Portland, Oregon

I don't feel like myself. What I loved doing before I don't
like to do anymore. This is confusing and scary for me.
Yoga used to calm me and now I am still angry afterwards.
Meeting with my girlfriends used to be fun and carefree; now
I am frustrated and sad when I get in my car to leave.

I've read the e-mails you sent me, but I can't remember your
words. I only hear in my head the things you say that hurt me.

I review our life together and all I can see is your betrayal.

Events that I used to cherish are now colored by your addiction.

My wedding ring means nothing. Our wedding photos are
dull. The house we live in is an empty shell. There is no us is
how I feel. And there is no me either. I don't know who I am.

Insecurity - Jacksonville, Florida

I will most likely ask a lot of questions. I'm now wondering what you wanted that I wasn't giving you. Especially if I think I was a really good wife, I may think there is no way to please you. If my self-esteem is stronger, I may believe that this really is about you and not about me. Instead of anger, I may feel disgust and repulsion. I may feel this either way.

If the images you were looking at look like me, I'm wondering if I was some sort of live replacement for them. I become not real. I become something you used and not a partner, friend, confidant, or love.

If the images you were looking at don't look like me, I think that your true desire is something different, especially if you have made references to me losing weight, or changing my hair color or the way I dress or don't dress.

The kind of porn you were looking at affects me. Are you thinking of those images when we are having sex? Do you want to have that kind of sex if the porn is different from our sex life? Have you ever enjoyed the sex we have together? I now wonder how often you use porn instead of being with me. I wonder if you use porn to avoid me, and I wonder what I have done or not done to cause this.

If your acting out has escalated to massage parlors or prostitutes, I am wondering how you find them, what you say to them, and how you pay them. I have so many questions. In the end, these questions are an attempt to take back my sanity. The questions are a way to try and keep myself safe. I thought I was safe with you, that I could trust you, and of course now, that is all shattered.

If you are now seeking help you are probably feeling better about your situation. You're "in recovery" is what they say and what you say. I'm still reeling from what has happened. I am trying to figure out what reality is now. So I ask questions. Sometimes I ask the same question many times over in a slightly different way. Sometimes the way I ask the question has sarcasm or contempt to it. I'm not really happy when I am this way. I don't feel good about myself in this space. But I feel even worse about what happened.

Sometimes I will wake up in the middle of the night with a new question. Sometimes my questions make sense, sometimes they don't. When you answer with "I don't know," this frustrates me even though the books and therapists say that you really don't know because you were in some dissociated state, and a piece of me doesn't believe this. I think you are making excuses. I think you don't really want to tell me the truth.

Sometimes I have put pieces together for myself. I have realized a time you were distant and did something like buy me jewelry or take me on vacation, and then I know it was when you broke off an affair, or started an affair, or your acting out had escalated in some way. Sometimes I have put another piece in the timeline and realized you acted out when our child was born or when you encouraged me to go out at night or told me it would be good to take a job that caused me to travel more. So I barrage you with questions. In some way it helps to know the truth. It makes me feel less crazy and more in control of my own mind and sanity.

And underneath all the questions are a couple of key questions. Why did you do this? How could you not be thinking of me when you were

doing this? And can you stop, did you stop,
how can I be sure this won't happen again?

I Need Help – Syracuse, New York

I think you think I've been the stronger one between the two of us. Maybe that was right once, but not anymore. For the first time I'm realizing I need help. You are feeling better and you are convinced it will never happen again. I'm not so sure. In fact, I don't know what to think or feel. I want to talk with some of my friends, but you say that will embarrass you or that you really don't want anyone to know.

So I feel I'm going crazy. I can't keep this to myself. I need help and you have been the one I have turned to all through our relationship. I can't turn to you now. As much as I would like to do that, I can't.

I also feel like no one can understand what I am going through. One therapist suggested I wear sexy lingerie, the couple's therapist we saw couldn't hear my distress, and I don't dare tell my family or they will hate you. Maybe I want that, but maybe I don't.

I don't know where to turn for help.

I Can't – Pierre, South Dakota

My sister says to leave you

I can't

My therapist says I should take care of myself

I can't

My pastor says to forgive you

I can't

My doctor says I should take time

I can't

I can't

I can't

Distrust – Cincinnati, Ohio

I think you know I don't trust you when it comes to telling the truth. What I'm trying to tell you is that I don't trust you with anything. Not money, not our children, not getting the right kind of bread from the grocery store. And yet you have the colossal nerve to argue with me because I have taken money out of our joint account and put it into my own account. You are surprised that I have taken my passport and hidden it. You think I am crazy for taking my family heirlooms to a storage locker. You are incensed that I would dare to do this! I can't believe that you don't get how your actions have put everything you say and do into question.

Let me try to explain how my mind is working right now. I have thoughts that you have a secret family. My mind is wondering if on all your business trips to San Diego you now have a complete other life there; another wife who you are also lying to. I have completely trusted you with our finances. Now I am wondering how you really spent your work bonuses. How much money have you spent on jewelry or trips with someone else?

My main goal right now is to keep myself safe. I have always thought I was safe with you. I am trying to patch up my security net because you ripped it to pieces.

What's Wrong with This Picture? - Mobile, Alabama

We've been seeing a new couple's therapist, and I'm really hopeful that she can help us. But she keeps asking me what my part is in all of this. I'm having a very difficult time staying in the room, mentally and physically, when this happens. Of course I have wondered what I could have done to make things better. I try to be engaged with the therapy but then I look over at you and is it smugness I see? Somehow I feel the tables have turned and now I'm the one who is under the microscope. This feels very, very wrong.

If – Evanston, Illinois

I'm trying to figure out all these ways to make sure you won't do "it" again.

If I have sex whenever you want.

If I stay angry with you.

If I try to not make you mad.

If I can make you happy.

Will this work? Is there anything at all I can do so you won't cheat on me?

Everyone I talk to says this is not my fault. Some say I have no control over you. Some say I have to let you figure this out. I can't let go of the possibility that if I can just DO something that you will be ok.

My mind goes to other ideas. What if we moved? Maybe if we went to Florida like we have been planning things will be different. What if I start working full-time like you have been complaining about. Would that fix things? And then I'm told that I can't fix it; I can't fix you. I'm used to making things better and finding ways to make what's wrong right. I've done this my whole life! I don't know how to do things any different.

Fragile – Washington, D.C.

I want to scream "Handle with Care"! Of course I don't even bother to try and communicate with you anymore. You just don't get it! No matter what I say, no matter what I do, you can't seem to understand and you don't act as if you care.

This fragility I've felt recently has really always been there, I've just had to cover it up over the years. I remember being teased as a kid and I learned to change my ways so that wouldn't happen. I can recall loving my doll and my brother cutting her long silky hair. My mom didn't punish him, and I learned not to show what my true likes and loves were ever again. The day my uncle came into my bedroom and touched me was also a day I learned to shut down, toughen up, protect and hide pieces of myself.

I thought with you I could learn to trust. I opened up to you more than I did to anyone else. That's one reason this all hurts so much. There's a voice inside my head that says, "You see? You can never trust anyone." I've tried to argue what seems like forever with those words. I've tried to believe that there are people who are kind and loving, who can accept me for who I am. I don't want to harden into a piece of steel. I know I can heal and move on, see and hear that there is love in the world and that I am worthy of that. However, for this moment, I feel the roots of my pain anchoring me into ice. I feel, if a strong wind blew, I would shatter into a million pieces.

Girls - Ashville, Washington

I thought pornography was okay. When you would watch it I just thought this is something all guys do. When you wanted to try something with me that you saw on the Internet, I thought it was harmless, something new to bring into our sex life. I never really thought about the girls and women in the videos. I thought this was a choice I wouldn't make, but no harm done.

Today I'm thinking differently. I think of all those girls. I think of myself as a girl. I go back and forth from thinking of them as sluts and whores to innocent, uneducated young women coerced into having sex in front of a camera. I've been reading that many of these women have been sexually abused when they were young. I've read they need to get drunk or high before they film.

And then I think of our little girl. I can't understand how you could watch those women do those things and not think of our daughter. I wonder how watching all that pornography has distorted the way you see women, all women.

Insanity – Jackson, Mississippi

There's a side of me that I don't recognize. This piece of me seems to pretend that you and I have a relationship. I hear my voice say to people, "Sam and I are going to take separate vacations this year, but that's good because I really like travelling by myself." Another example is I'll be trying to plan a dinner with friends and name all the dates you can't be there. "Sam has a business trip that week. Or, Sam doesn't like to go out on Sundays." It feels like the equivalent of a child saying Mommy doesn't want me to eat a cookie before dinner. My voice sounds young and almost pleading but with a certain assertion that I know you better than others. Which, of course, as your wife, I should, so it gets confusing.

I think I need to change this. This is the codependency that all the books say I have if I am with an addict. I've fought against this idea forever. How could I be codependent? I'm so strong and independent? I have my own job, my own money, and my own friends. I couldn't possibly put your needs before mine! But that voice.....betrays me. My feelings when I am in that place, betray me. If I am honest, I will do a lot to make a relationship work. The problem is I really don't believe you are working as hard as I am because if you were working on it, I wouldn't have to be making excuses for you, now would I?

I Should Have Known – Santa Fe, New Mexico

In the midst of all my anger is an embarrassment and
self-admonishment that somehow I should have known.
I feel really stupid. Now, as I look back, there were so
many clues. That night you said you were in Denver
with your friend, who you never socialize with,
was when you were with one of those women.
I don't even have to ask you now; I just know. I feel
pathetic because I asked you to bring me home
a Caesar salad, which you dutifully did,
after having dinner with her.

There were other events. I couldn't understand why
you didn't want to stand in the family picture at my
cousin's wedding. You didn't want me to come with
you to Los Angeles over spring break; said it would
be boring. It's the beach! And then when I did go,
there was the strange phone call with a lovely
woman's voice on the other end asking for you by first
and last name. You denied you knew who this was, and
at that moment, I knew something was very, very
wrong, but I so wanted to believe you. I wanted to believe
that you wouldn't do anything to hurt me
or our marriage. I've resisted admitting that I was
in denial, that on some level I knew. I *did* know.

I just couldn't face the enormity of the truth. I couldn't wrap my head around what this would mean for me, for you and for our family.

Forgiveness – Charleston, South Carolina

You are asking me to forgive you. I want to, but I don't want to lie. Forgive and forget or forgive but don't forget? My defenses are so high that I don't dare forgive you. I understand more each day about what this is and what happened to you and to us. My head can put this into perspective, but my heart refuses to let go of the insanity of it all and the hurt.

Forgive you. What if you have a "slip" or a "relapse," what then? The books say you probably will and if I forgive you once, will I have to forgive you once again, twice again, twenty times? "How much can I take?" I ask myself. What is fair – to you and to me – to keep a marriage together? How many relapses must I suffer through before I'm irretrievably broken?

Forgive you. For give. For the sake of giving. I'm starting to wonder what I've gotten in giving. I'm wondering if I gave too much over the course of our relationship. People talk about not controlling you. I'm thinking I didn't control you enough. Maybe if I had been more vigilant you wouldn't have done this.

I can't forgive you. Not now. Maybe later. It's too big. I'd be forgiving something I can't even understand. I'd be saying everything is okay when it obviously is not. I need you to forgive me for not being able to forgive you. Maybe we can start there.

Our life together – Chicago, Illinois

I keep wondering where you found the time and energy to do all this acting out. We're together almost all the time. When we're not together, you're at work. My mind is trying to figure out how and when you could have done these things. My mind flutters between all the great times we have had together, and how our entire relationship was a lie!

I'm so sad. I was living one reality and you were living another. I have no idea what I mean to you. I think you were with me only because I paid half the mortgage, was a good mother and kept the house clean. I think you obviously didn't stay with me for the sex; you were getting that elsewhere, whether that was porn or prostitution or an affair. You didn't stay with me because I made you happy; otherwise you wouldn't have gone outside our relationship to spend time with other women! These are all thoughts I can't help having. I know the sex addiction thing says you were only with those women to have sex, but I was willing to be sexual with you! I wanted to try different things and grow closer to you intimately. WHY did you have to do that with other women? If you were using porn, that's the same as having sex with someone else. Those pictures of women were taking you away from me. You would rather masturbate to those images than have intercourse with me. Do you have any idea how that makes me feel?

Our life together will never be the same. I'm thinking of getting rid of the bed, the living room chairs and re-painting the house. If, IF, you had a woman in our home, we may need to sell the house too. We may need to sell the house anyway. I don't know if I can live here anymore. I may demand you get rid of certain clothes, have you change your cologne, get rid of hobbies depending on how the betrayal occurred. Maybe you have to find another job. I may want an entire new wardrobe since what I was wearing wasn't good enough. If I clothe shopped sales racks, I may feel resentful and angry and may want nice, expensive clothes now. If you bought women gifts or jewelry, I may want you to buy me the same thing, only nicer; and then the next minute not want any of it. I expect you to sit beside me on this roller-coaster ride. I need you to not argue, not tell me I'm crazy, not shut down, and not spiral into shame. For all the time you have spent over the years in your addiction, you can help me through this time of emotional hell.

What Can You Do? – Seattle, Washington

"What can I do" you ask. You can be patient. You can tell me you aren't going to leave. You can tell me you aren't going to push me and that you know you have hurt me.

You can think of new ways to show you love me. What you said or did for me before is now a lie and if you did that same thing for another woman, that gesture is now polluted. You say you are just trying to be yourself, but you've shared yourself with others when it should have been just me. Every overture needs to be absolutely pure now. Nothing can be rehearsed or rote, unconscious or glib.

And I think *how the hell can he do this? If this is addiction and an intimacy disorder, how can he do what I need him to do?* At these times I get incredibly sad. At these times you ask what you can do, or you may seem hopeless yourself, or get angry, or withdraw. This is the worst thing you can do. You need to be patient.

Anger – Detroit, Michigan

Really? You really are getting angry with me? How dare you, in that aggressive demanding stance, say I'm doing something wrong! You were the one who went outside of our marriage. You were the one who betrayed our relationship. And now you are saying you are angry because I bought our daughter a cell phone before asking you if that was okay. Who the hell do you think you are? What makes you think you have the right to make ANY decisions about our family anymore? I'm done being intimidated by you. I'm done being bullied by you. I'm thinking I am done with you.

PART FOUR:

Making Decisions

Pain is inevitable. Suffering is optional.

Buddha

There comes a time where you know with certainty that you will be okay. You will survive. For some people this happens quickly after the time of Discovery and for others it is much longer. Some describe this feeling as landing on a lily pad in a pond of still water; there's stability, but it is not completely grounded. If you move too suddenly, your balance will be disrupted, so you learn to move carefully. You are able to look at all the situations around you differently. At this stage you realize you have a lot of decisions to make, although you may not know all the answers quite yet. And you experience a calm in the storm.

Patience – Louisville, Kentucky

I love you. But my patience is wearing thin. I think of our life together and our marriage. Every time there was an event that could have brought us closer together, you retreated into a distant place that I couldn't reach. I always wondered where you would go. At first I thought of you as sort of mysterious. Sometimes I saw your silence as something of a challenge. If I could reach you, connect with you, then I'd have accomplished something special. I don't think you realize, but I spent a lot of time thinking of ways to get closer to you. Sometimes it was arranging a special dinner date. Sometimes it was conceding and watching TV shows or movies that I knew you'd like, but I didn't. Sometimes it was having sex when I didn't want to. But I did. I did all these things to try and be close to you.

The idea, in spite of everything that I tried and did, that you would go to other women, whether in pictures or real life, is beyond my comprehension. I ask myself if there is anything else I could have done? And then I come up with I just wasn't good enough. Not good enough in bed, at parties, with your family. And so I cling to our children because they are my only refuge now. I want to tell them how awful you are. I want to show them how you have betrayed our family. I want to make them believe you should be punished for a long, long time. Our children, in some ways, are becoming *my* children. And then there are days, minutes, moments when I wish I had never had children with you. I worry that my boy will be like you. I worry that my girl will marry someone who hurts her.

And then, unexpectedly, you will tell me you are going to your 12-step meeting, or that you were tempted in some way and resisted. I don't understand how these meetings work, and I don't yet trust you are where you say you are. You've lied to me so many times. Yet, there it is sneaking up from some centered place in my soul - hope. I can't believe it when it pops up. I'm hoping and praying that those meetings work. I'm holding my breath hoping your therapist can help. I'm begging the universe to please, please have something happen so you will change.

This is why I ask so many questions when you come in the door. This is why I question you over and over again about the past. I have no compass to navigate these waters. I am a ship without a rudder in the middle of a storm, and I am so scared. I feel I am on the brink of losing everything; my family, my marriage, my sanity, my faith, my life. I try to let you not see this. I try to not let anyone see this. I've always been a strong woman, but I am now broken in a way I never thought possible.

So I am trying to be patient. I'm watching and waiting and willing to stay, although I said I would leave. I hope I am not being a complete idiot. I look at our kids and I know that they are the main reason I stay.

Taking Note – St. Paul, Minnesota

There's a piece of me that is thinking that I
don't want to do certain things anymore. When
I see the laundry not getting done unless I do
it, I'm starting to take note. When I realize
that if I don't make dinner that you order a
pizza, under the dullness is awareness.

I'm also looking at all the time I spent doing
things I didn't care about. Also I've participated in
events and gave time to people that I didn't like
or with whom I felt awkward or uncomfortable.
I never liked our neighbors, and I continued to
have them over for dinner and drinks. I hated
going to your parents' house for holidays. If I
remember, so did you. Why did we continue to go?

My therapist gave me a book on co-dependency.
I am reading a little of it; a page or two from
time to time. I hate the word co-dependency. I'm
NOT co-dependent. And I'm wondering if I have
given too much. I always thought that's what part
of being a good wife or partner was all about.

I Don't Know What This Is – Hot Springs, Arkansas

I've been thinking a lot about why I can't understand
what has happened to you and what is happening
to you. I just can't get my head around it. I heard
a story that when Christopher Columbus sailed to
Hispaniola, the natives could not "see" their huge ships.
The theory goes that if you have never experienced
something, or it is not in your perception of reality, that
you won't register it. Whether this story is true or not,
it resonates with me. How can I possibly be able to
relate or understand this thing, this sex addiction thing
when I have never had any experience with it? How
could I have recognized it? My family has not had any
addiction. My previous boyfriends haven't been addicted.
I don't have any kind of compulsivity to speak of.

So it's going to take me some time to take in what
this is. I need to think in a new paradigm. For me,
everything you talk about, from your meetings to phrases
you are using, is all new. And I, of course, wonder if
this is real, just like the natives who couldn't believe
what gods or devils were coming onto their land.

Trust – Nashville, Tennessee

I am hearing from you that you want me to trust you. This is hard for me because I did trust you for so very long. Even when I was suspicious, I still believed you. Often you said you were at work, meeting a friend to go to dinner, or going to the grocery store, but actually you were going off to act out. I don't say this to guilt trip you. I now know how terrible you feel. I'm saying this to remind you of all the time I invested in "keeping the faith."

Pretending – Durango, Colorado

I've been kidding myself in some way. I've allowed lies and half-truths into my life. I can't pretend that you were the woman I thought you were. I can't pretend this didn't happen. Somehow I got sucked into continuing to believe that you were an honest person and had integrity. Based on my love for you, I decided to believe you even when I had suspicions that things you said didn't make sense.

I would like some sort of explanation that makes sense of what has become of you. I've rifled through all the possibilities. Is it me? Is it you? Are you bi-polar? Or borderline? An alcoholic? A sex addict? Friends throw these words out to me, offering some reason why you are doing this to me and our family. All I know is a piece of me cannot continue to live this way. You are not stopping and this is killing me.

Mixed Up – Cheyenne, Wyoming

I'm really mixed up. You were really good at convincing me to do things during sex that I thought were okay, but now I'm weirded out by those things. I think you made a lot of strange things seem normal, you know? I feel all scared and insecure with myself and my body, and I never felt this way before you. That sounds mean, I know, but I just keep thinking about not knowing everything you were doing and then the sex we had and now feeling gross that I didn't listen to my intuition when I knew things were getting strange. But I felt we had such chemistry. Now I know there was all that bad stuff going on and that I didn't know anything for sure.

If we split up and I'm with someone else, I'm hoping that all this crap doesn't carry over. I hope that it is only you that has made me this way, and that if I am with someone who cares about me, they will bring me back to some normal place; but I'm also afraid I'm damaged forever. I'm upset for the things we did do, and upset for the things we didn't do. I knew I should have left you, and I don't know why I stayed so long, and I still don't understand what was real between us and what was a lie.

And now I'm really confused because I thought you loved me, but how could anyone really love someone and do what you did? I really do get that you were and are really messed up, especially with what happened to you when you were a kid. No one knows about the sexual stuff with your cousin but me, and I really think you should tell your family what happened. Maybe if you get healthy we could still be together. Then again, I don't know if I can ever forgive you.

So anyway, that's all I have to say except that I still do love you and care about you and I hope you can get better somehow.

Unsure – Baton Rouge, Louisiana

I want to leave but I also want to stay.
I cling onto the small hope that you will
get better. I grasp onto the idea that you
really are sick. But then the memories and
thoughts in my head rush up, and I see the
pictures you looked at for years. I ask myself,
how can I be blonde instead of brunette
because that is what I think you want? How can
I be 130 pounds instead of 160? And then I
remember that I did work out, and I did lose
weight. I changed my hair and bought different
clothes, and yet you still went and did what
you did. When I think this through, all the
old pain comes back, and I realize that
nothing I did or didn't do really mattered.

I still am unsure if we should be together.
And I don't know how to ask you, and I am too
weak sometimes to risk hearing your answer.
But what I need is for you to tell me I am
the only woman for you. I need you to tell
me you love everything about me. I need to
hear that those women were ugly. That you
realize those women you were looking at were

sad, manipulated, tortured souls and that they are not the kind of woman you want to be with.

Can You Be Honest With Me? – Billings, Montana

You are still telling lies. You say that you are sober and strangely enough on some level I believe you. But then you lie about having taken the dog out! Why would you not tell me the truth about something so basic?

When you can't be honest about small, simple things, how can I keep believing that you are telling the truth about the bigger more important piece; your sobriety?

Please, please figure out why you keep doing this.

Don't Tell – Raleigh, North Carolina

I've kept your secret until now because you
asked me to, but I can't keep this up anymore.
I have to talk to people who are important to
me about what's happened. Your mother keeps
asking me if everything is alright. She knows
something is wrong. My sister is wondering
why I haven't been calling her. My friends
don't know why I've been avoiding them.

Can you please tell your parents? And can you
do that so they will not blame me? Please use words
like "addiction" and "this isn't Kathy's fault, it's
mine." If they want to talk to me, I need them
to not be defensive or talk about how this is
hurting them. What I really need is for them just
to ask me what they can do to help, even
though I may not have an answer right now.
I need to know they care about how this
has affected me, too. Knowing your family
as I do, this could be asking too much.

I have to tell my friends and family. I am willing
to talk to you about what I should say. I get that
this is shameful and embarrassing to you.

I'm going to ask you to work that out with your therapist, sponsor, whoever. I can't stand holding this secret for any longer.

Gravity – Houston, Texas

As much as I have read all the books, talked to my friends, gone to therapy, and talked to you, I really have not understood what all of this means. This afternoon it hit me. You really are a sex addict. I also started to feel the enormity of what this means. No matter how much you work at this, you will always be a sex addict. You may be recovering but still an addict. I need to ask myself if I can be in a committed relationship with someone who is addicted. This is a serious question, perhaps the most serious one I've had to face.

My Life – Concord, New Hampshire

What have I done with my life? I feel I've given so much to you and our family. Why? Why did I give so much?

Quiet – Little Rock, Arkansas

It's midnight. The kids are all in bed and this is the hour when I can stop and have time for myself. I've asked you to leave and give me my space. I struggle with this decision; however, I know it is right because when you come back home; I feel my anxiety increase, and the wall I let down comes back up again. I don't want it to come up again; it just does.

During the day I focus on having a happy face for the children. I don't want them to see me sad. I want to be there for them. It's hardest on the youngest because I know I can't give him what I have given his brothers and sisters. I wonder how this will go for him later on in his life. I wonder and fear he will hate me because I can't love him like I want.

In the quiet of the night I cry. I cry for me, for our children, for you and for us. I wonder how we can stay married. I wonder how other people survive this.

Sex - Portland, Maine

I'm a little mixed up about sex right
now. Part of me wants to have sex with
you because I'm afraid that if I don't,
you'll act out. Part of me doesn't want to
stop having sex with you because that is
the main way I felt connected to you.

BUT, when we do have sex, I'm thinking about
the girls you were looking at on the Internet.
And I can't help but compare myself to them.
I was never that confident about my sexuality
or my looks and now I can't help but think
that you want them and not me. "Why do you
really want to be with me?" I think. There's
not anything you can do or say for me to
believe you now. Sometimes I think about being
with another man just to bring my confidence
up. Sometimes I think of having an affair
to get back at you. But I know this will
only hurt our relationship more than ever.

There are times when we are intimate and I
believe I'm okay, that I'm over those horrible
feelings. And then we have a big fight. My

therapist tells me this is my way of creating distance and I don't trust you yet. She says my body isn't ready. How can I be in this place of wanting to be close to you, terrified to let you touch me, and numbing out, when I used to be thrilled by your attention? I can't say much of this to you. I don't want you to blame me or have an excuse to act out. I do blame myself for your turning away from me.

I suppose I need to know for sure that you are no longer acting out in order to be intimate with you. I need to know, somehow, that if I really am not comfortable with some of the sex you asked for, that that is completely okay. I need to know that you love me and that our sex life is not the only reason we are together, and that you want me and want to be with me even if we never had sex again.

I don't want to be just another vagina to you.

Anniversaries–Des Moines, Iowa

I sometimes will be doing fine. I'll feel that life is better and that we have put this whole thing behind us. And then, all of a sudden, a wave of despair or anxiety washes over me. When this happens I either go into a rage or a depression. I didn't know what it was until someone mentioned this thing called "anniversaries." This is when my body and unconscious mind will remember a time or place or thing associated with your acting out behavior, I'm told.

The other day I was sitting in the living room waiting for the children to come home. It was the first day of spring when the weather changes from snow to icy rain. I watched as the windows became streaked with water, and I suddenly burst out crying. I had no idea why. I talked with a friend and she reminded me that two years ago was when this all began. My conscious mind had forgotten the connection but apparently some part of me remembered.

This sort of thing happens at other times too. When our wedding anniversary nears, I become sad. If I try to push away or ignore the feelings, they only get stronger. Rationally, this makes no sense. I know you are working hard, and I believe you are trying not to fall back into your old ways. And I still have these times of unpredictable darkness.

The other day you and I took a different route home and we drove past your old workplace. I grew very quiet and snapped at you about the music being too loud. I now realize seeing the building you went to every day and where you were seeing that woman makes my whole body scream with anger and fear.

I had hoped with time this would go away. We had to get rid of clothes, furniture, gifts and anything associated with your infidelity. I don't regret that. I am hoping we can still stay in this same city, but I wonder sometimes, if leaving and moving somewhere completely different would help. I don't want to keep feeling like this.

Selfish – Wichita, Kansas

My mama raised me to be kind, considerate, caring,
and understanding. These were what a proper girl
was. I was told to be selfish was inappropriate and
that I should never, never act <u>this</u> way. So when I
was angry – I stuffed that away, and tried harder to
be kind and loving just like Mother Mary was when I
saw her sweet face in church on Sunday mornings.

Now I'm being told this is <u>not </u>what I should be
doing. Think of <u>yourself.</u> What do <u>you</u> need,
what do <u>you</u> want? This just was not the way
I was raised! But I will try. If this is what is
going to heal me and help heal us, I will do my
best, even though it feels awfully selfish.

Innocence Lost – Arlington, Virginia

When I was a little girl I had a dream of marrying a man who was fun and charming and who would take care of me. I wouldn't admit this to anyone else, but you were that man! And I have had some bad things happen to me, but the way I was raised I knew I could handle just about anything. You of all people know I have had struggles. This experience, though, has made me a different person. I realize I have to grieve for the loss of the innocence I had about love, romance, men, and relationships

I feel robbed and shaken awake at the same time. I am hoping this won't lead to my being jaded about you or love. I want to fall in love again, hopefully with you, but, if not, with another man. I liked having a bright, cheerful view on romance, honeymoons, and marriage. I want that again.

PART FIVE:

Moving On

In order for the light to shine so brightly, the darkness must be present.

- Francis Bacon

Healing comes. We realize this journey has not been consistent. Sometimes the process has felt as if we move two steps forward and one to two steps back. Strange concepts enter into our awareness like gratitude, acceptance, and a razor sharp clarity. We know now that we can do more than survive; we can thrive. Life from now on might be very different from the past. Some may decide to leave their partners, some may decide to stay and either way losses are grieved and there are insightful, meaningful lessons learned.

Worth It - Pittsburgh, Pennsylvania

I have twenty or so years left in my life. You are an
alcoholic and a sex addict. I'm sixty years old, which is
hard to believe. I feel sorry for you and I feel sorry for me.
You know I have lost a lot of relationships through all of
this. Our daughters won't talk to either of us; they don't
understand. I divorced you. I had to divorce you and now
we are planning to elope and re-marry. I think I have one
friend who has stuck by through it all and although she is
supportive, she has held her tongue many times I am sure.

I love you. I have always loved you. And I always will.
Of course you have also done all the right things. We
have a therapist who knows sex addiction and I trust
him to know if you are bull-shitting. I have done a
lot of work that I didn't want to do to know what my
boundaries are and how to set them. You have stopped all
your nonsense and are acting like a real husband. I had
to let go of you to find myself. What a pair we make!

A Glimmer of Hope – Boston, Massachusetts

I'm not crying anymore. I can't believe it. And dare I say I felt happy today. Well not happy, but I wasn't scared or mad or sad or numb. That's good, isn't it? A bit of relief from the onslaught? I don't even know why but I'm grateful. Somehow, some way, I know I'm going to be okay. THAT is a miracle. It's strange. It's not this intense realization or an exciting event. It's a subtle, deep, grounded knowing. It's like the first day of spring when the air suddenly changes, but it's barely perceptible, and you know winter is over. It's the feeling you have the night after a fever breaks and you know the illness has passed and you can sleep and eat again.

I'm a little surprised. I didn't think I could recover. Yet here I am thinking about the future, making plans, calling people I haven't connected with for months. I'm breathing a sigh of relief. I'm going to survive.

Discerning – Denver, Colorado

I've been told that as you recover from your addiction, you will be a changed man. When I ask if the parts of you that I don't like, have never liked, will change, no one can give me a straight answer. I never liked the way you dressed. Will that change? I was irritated when you ate with your mouth open. Will you stop doing that? You would go to the bathroom and leave the door open. I hated that. So which one is you and which one is the addict?

I'm coming to the realization that even if you stop using pornography; these other pieces of you that I have tolerated over the years will still be there, maybe. I don't think I want to have these as a part of my life anymore. When I hear myself say this, I feel as if I'm being cruel in some way. Funny, after all the lying and deception, that I should feel mean about stating the truth.

I still think, despite everything, that you are a good father. This gives me more hope that we can be separated and that our children will be alright. I don't think they mind your idiosyncrasies. That's a good thing.

Just for Today – Birmingham, Alabama

I had the strangest feeling today as I was driving and I thought something was really wrong. What I realized is that I had this overwhelming feeling of calm. And I realized I haven't felt that in so long that I didn't trust it because I didn't recognize it. On the one side my body was so relieved and thankful and on the other side my mind was saying, "it is dangerous to relax; it is dangerous not to feel on guard." So I have two feelings; the first is I'm very happy that I can have this experience back again of being in my body and being in the world and not having to think so much and not having to worry. I can look at the sky and breathe in the air and just be alive. On the other hand, I am sad that I have been hurting for so long. That I've had to be in a place of not being connected, of being scared and unsure, and that makes me feel bad. But for today I'm just going to take a breath and do something simple for myself, something to mark this amazing shift that is mine today.

Leaving – Hartford, Connecticut

I would have done just about anything for you...I have never trusted anyone the way I trusted you, with my money, secrets, fear, and success. I miss believing you thought I was the best thing that ever happened to you. I miss being certain I was the only one you would marry. I miss the way we worked together to create a family. I miss supporting each other in our hopes, dreams and disappointments. You were everything to me and I didn't want to be with anyone else.

I miss our early years of beautiful cards, glorious holidays, celebrating each other. I miss the way we would work together on whichever house we were living in. I miss our cat and dog family.

I also miss the innocent side of you I saw when we first met. You seemed insulated from the world in a very soft, tender way. You hadn't experienced crime, big cities, economic insecurity, or racial tensions. Little did I know your protection from it created some need for it!

This part of life with you is now part of a greater history. It is one piece of a much larger puzzle.

I am glad I didn't spend any more time trying to force you into a relationship that you no longer wished to be a part of. Some would have wished to be taken out earlier; I am not one of them. I feel the twists and turns we executed, like trying to complete a Rubic's cube, were the exact right number to end.

On The Other Side – Kearney, Nebraska

Thank you. You've decided you aren't an addict and you have no problems regarding pornography or your sexual behavior. And now I have to leave. The decision isn't mine to make. You made it for both of us. You've made the choice and with the last shred of self-confidence I have, I'm ending the relationship.

This is a strange place. I have a wide, open space in front of me. I don't know what's ahead and I can't look behind. Usually my head would be racing with thoughts and feelings but not today; not now. I imagine this was what it was like years ago when parents would arrange marriages or young men would be called into war to be soldiers. There's a relief that I am not in control, but a sadness, too, at what I have lost. My wish is that we both will find peace. Good bye.

Reflection - Madison, Wisconsin

My father died shortly after our Florida
vacation. My mother phoned while we were
still in the airport. That night we stayed up
talking until three in the morning. I felt
so close to you and I needed you so much.
Shortly thereafter you asked me to support you
in taking a sales job with more travelling.
Why didn't I say "no"? Somehow I told myself
that this was helping you and us. How did I
miss that you were only taking jobs that were
to Asian countries? Somewhere in the back
of my mind a voice said, "There's something
very wrong. This is more than just wanting to
expand his career." I shut out those thoughts.

When you called and said your car was in
an accident and "You must be the most
important thing to me still because
you were the last thing I was thinking
of." I thought, "That's sweet, but what
else would you be thinking of?"

There were lots of doubts I had during
those years. I tried to protect and steel

myself for what I thought I knew would come. I could have never predicted the magnitude of your behaviors. But I've grown through this time. I've learned to trust my instinct again. I'm learning the real you from the addict. Before when Sly (my name for your addict) would pop up, I would just be confused. Now I see him so clearly and can just hang up the phone or walk away.

Staying – Trenton, New Jersey

I'm not going to divorce you. I couldn't do that to you or me or our family. What you have done is the past and you are saying you will never hurt me again, and I believe you.

So we will move forward. You've cried and started going to meetings; you're reading books and telling me how awful your life has been. I truly feel sorry for you. I know this is not the life you want.

I know you can succeed at whatever you put your mind to. I pray to God that you will be healed and that you can find peace and comfort. I love you.

Suspicion – Virginia Beach, Virginia

I knew something was wrong; I just couldn't put my finger on it. The way you would look sometimes when you came in the door. You started wanting different things sexually. You started shaving where you had not shaved before. All of this was confusing and disturbing. Our lives were so busy I, frankly, didn't have time to give it much thought. When I think back on some of it I realize my stomach was tense or my head felt strange. It is only now that I know, and they say hindsight is 20/20.

I want to say I wished I'd known sooner, but I would be lying. If I'd known sooner we wouldn't have had our children, or have had this home. If I had known sooner who knows what would have happened with our lives? As angry as I am that this has happened, I still want to make our marriage work.

There are some that disagree with me. Some women feel they would not have had children with their sex addict husbands if they knew then what they know now. There are women who can't believe other women stay with their boyfriends even though they now know they have cheated. Still others say they are willing to stay IF the addiction is only to pornography.

I had a feeling; other women said they had no idea. Now, if I have "a feeling" again, I will definitely speak up. I expect you to be honest every time I ask, no matter what I ask or how many times.

Re-entering My Life – Colorado Springs, Colorado

I hadn't seen him in seven months and during that time my life started over. My concerns and worries and frustrations turned to normal things, like the long line at the bank or if Social Security would still be around when I turn 65. And then I started thinking that a decision would have to be made about where to hold that milestone birthday party.

My life – re-entered.

One Day at a Time – Scottsdale, Arizona

The strangest thing happened today. I woke up, had my
breakfast, fed the dog and went to work. It was a busy day. Lots
of surgeries and injuries. I spent the day nursing sick dogs and
angry cats. Kept me occupied. After work, I had dinner with
a girlfriend, and we had a lot of laughs. When I got home,
it struck me: I hadn't thought of you once all day long.

It's been a year, and I thought I'd never stop thinking
about you and the way you firebombed my life. For a
while, I ate, slept, and dreamed you. It seemed I'd never
get over it. But today I didn't think of you until now.

Maybe tomorrow I won't think of you at all. In the
meantime, I'm easing down the road to a life of my own.

A Poem called Hope – San Francisco, California

I am pulled between sanity, which
moves and flies forward,

And the insanity, that whirls with hope
for recovery and reconciliation.

This empty nest with shattered
eggshells and in-utero goo,

Of matted feathers, dirty and torn.

The wind blows the dried sticks and
twigs, the barren refuge, unsecured.

Staring past, I see birds busily collecting
– paper, grass, strewn nature objects.

They fly up – poking, placing,
picking in preparation,

Preparing a new home to cradle
and nurture newborns, again.

AFTERWORD

There are a few things I believe to be true when going through this experience. The first is that the person betrayed needs help and support. It doesn't matter how strong you have been in the past, you need the clarity and unconditional love of friends and family. Most likely you will find out quickly who is capable of being there for you at this confusing and critical time.

I also believe you need an experienced therapist who understands what you are going through and how to guide you through this. I've had too many clients come to me and say, "My therapist is looking at me, telling me I'm doing great and she/he can't believe what I've been through. They seem overwhelmed by my situation. If they can't handle this, how can I!" Finding a therapist who works with trauma and understands sex addiction is the best combination.

Trusting someone new will be hard, especially right after discovery. You may go through seeing more than one therapist, which is not optimal, but sometimes happens. My suggestion is that you set boundaries with whomever you begin to work with. This may sound like "I don't want to talk about my family of origin." Or "I don't believe this has anything to do with me. I just need to talk about him." If the therapist can't respect that boundary, this is a good indication they can't meet you where you are at, and it may be time to find another clinician. In time, after the trauma has settled, you will have many questions about yourself and how you ended up in a relationship with an addict. This may be months or years down the road. This is a process, which takes up to four years if both addict and partner are getting appropriate treatment, and more if treatment is delayed or not sought at all.

The main certification program in sex addiction is through an organization called IITAP, International Institute for Trauma and Addiction Professionals. IITAP offers a list of certified sex addiction therapists throughout the world. The web site is www.iitap.com. You will be able to find a CSAT in your area.

Partner Assessment

1. Has your husband, wife, or significant other, been more irritable, depressed, angry and/or distant?

2. Has his/her behavior changed so that he/she is leaving the house early, coming home late or absent during the day where normally he/she would be home or answering phone calls or texts?

3. Is he suddenly asking for different sexual behaviors?

4. Has she been distant or uninterested in you sexually?

5. Is he lying about or hiding his pornography use?

6. Are you feeling compelled to check credit card or phone bill statements?

7. Are you feeling you need to check e-mail accounts and/or web-site histories?

8. Do you find yourself normalizing a less than satisfying relationship?

9. Do you find yourself making excuses for him?

10. Have you felt more like a mother or father than a lover?

11. Are you desperate for any type of affection from your partner?

12. If you are in couples counseling, do you feel he/she is conning the therapist?

13. Do you feel frightened or intimidated to set limits with him/her?

14. Are you afraid to ask for your needs to be met?

15. Do you now find yourself jealous or uncomfortable with your partner's behavior around the opposite sex?

16. Are you compromising yourself to keep the relationship?

17. Do you feel you are going crazy?

18. Do you feel your reality is surreal?

19. Are you eating more or eating foods to feel better?

20. Or do you find you are so anxious that you can't eat?

21. Do you find yourself working extra hard to connect to your partner?

22. Do you feel something is very wrong in your relationship with your partner?

If you answered "yes" to four or more questions, I would suggest consulting with someone who specializes in sex addiction for greater clarity and further education. You can also read the web sites and material cited in the resources section of this book.

Where to go for help

12-Step programs are a cornerstone of breaking free from compulsive behavior.

For sex addiction you can find meetings at ....
Sexaholics Anonymous (SA)
www.sa.org
866-424-8777
Sex Addicts Anonymous(SAA)
www.saa-recovery.org
800-477-8191
Sex and Love Addicts Anonymous(SLAA)
www.slaafws.org
210-828-7900

For alcoholism...
Alcoholics Anonymous (AA)
www.aa.org
212-870-3400

For drug addiction....

Narcotics Anonymous

www.na.org

818-773-9999

Marijuana Anonymous

www.marijuana-anonymous.org

800-766-6779

For support if your spouse is addicted to sex or porn at .....

Codependents of sex addicts(COSA)

www.cosa-recovery.org

763-537-6904

S-Anon

www.sanon.org

800-210-8141

If you are both involved in 12-step programs...

Recovering Couples Anonymous (RCA)

www.recovering-couples.org

510-663-2312

Additional Resources

A.A. Big Book by The Augustine Fellowship

As We Understood by Al-Anon

Courage to Change by Al-Anon

One Day at a Time in Al-Anon by Al-Anon

Opening Our Hearts; Transforming Our Losses by Al-Anon

Reflections of Hope by S-Anon

S-Anon Twelve Steps by S-Anon

Working the S-Anon Program by S-Anon

The White Book by Sexaholics Anonymous

The Green Book by Sex Addicts Anonymous

Sex and Love Addicts Anonymous: The Basic Text for The Augustine Fellowship

If you would like to have more information about sex addiction the following books can be helpful. If you realize you are not remembering what you are reading, this just means you are still in trauma and that you may need to wait to be able to better retain the material.

Books Regarding Trauma

Waking The Tiger
By Peter Levine
Waking the Tiger normalizes the symptoms of trauma and the steps needed to heal them. The reader is taken on a guided tour of the subtle, yet powerful impulses that govern our responses to overwhelming life events. To do this, it employs a series of exercises that help us focus on bodily sensations. Through heightened awareness of these sensations trauma can be healed.

The Trauma Spectrum
By Robert Scaer
Our experiences of trauma sow the seeds of many persistent and misunderstood medical problems such as chronic fatigue syndrome and various maladies of the immune system. Because of our inadequate understanding of the relationship of mind and body in processing these traumas, many of us suffer needlessly from our exposure to life's traumas. Robert Scaer offers hope to those who wish to transform trauma and better understand their lives.

BrainSpotting: The Revolutionary New Therapy for Rapid and Effective Change

By David Grand

"Brainspotting lets the therapist and client participate together in the healing process," explains Dr. Grand. "It allows us to harness the brain's natural ability for self-scanning, so we can activate, locate, and process the sources of trauma and distress in the body." With *Brainspotting,* this pioneering researcher introduces an invaluable tool that can support virtually any form of therapeutic practice and greatly accelerate our ability to heal.

Getting Past Your Past: Take Control of Your Life with Self-Help Techniques from EMDR Therapy

By Francine Shapiro

Whether we've experienced small setbacks or major traumas, we are all influenced by memories and experiences we may not remember or don't fully understand. Getting Past Your Past offers practical procedures that demystify the human condition and empower readers looking to achieve real change. Shapiro, the creator of EMDR (Eye Movement Desensitization and Reprocessing), explains how our personalities develop and why we become trapped into feeling, believing and acting in ways that don't serve us.

Books for Partners of Sex Addicts

Your Sexually Addicted Spouse: How Partners Can Cope and Heal

by Barbara Steffens, Marsha Means

The authors lay out the case that 12-step programs for partners of sex addicts can be harmful in labeling the partner as a co-addict, or co-dependent, and that the pain that partners experience after discovery of their partner's behavior is best understood as a trauma that can have long lasting effects.

Mending A Shattered Heart: A Guide for Partners of Sex Addicts

By Stephanie Carnes, Ph.D.

A go-to guide covering important subjects such as whether to stay in the relationship or leave, when and how life gets better, how to set boundaries and what to say to the children.

Back From Betrayal: Recovering From His Affairs, Third Edition

By Jennifer P. Schneider

This is a new edition of a classic book for women and men whose spouses or partners have had multiple affairs or sex addiction problems. Dr. Schneider explains how 12-Step recovery programs can work for you, and provides straightforward guidance on how to find self-help groups and how to choose a therapist. The 2005 Third Edition is expanded and updated, with additional material for men whose partners have affairs, a chapter on cybersex and Internet affairs, information on disclosing secrets to one's partner and children, and updated medical information on sexually transmitted diseases.

Ready to Heal
By Kelly McDaniel
Help for those struggling in a relationship with a sex addict, facing their own sex addiction, obsessing about someone who doesn't want you, or looking for deeper understanding of romantic patterns. At its core, love and sex addiction is a longing for intimacy. Since love, connection, and sexual intimacy are basic human needs, healing addictive relationships prepares you to give and receive love in healthy ways. Part of being ready to heal is having faith that although you don't know what will happen, you are prepared to move forward on the journey.

Books about Sex Addiction

Out of the Shadows: Understanding Sexual Addiction
by Patrick Carnes, Ph.D.
The premier work on sex addiction, *Out of the Shadows* describes the danger signs, explains the dynamics and describes the consequences of sexual addiction and compulsivity. This book has practical wisdom and gives spiritual clarity.

In the Shadows of the Net: Breaking Free of Compulsive Online Sexual Behavior
by Patrick Carnes, David Delmonico, and Elizabeth Griffin.

As Internet usage has exploded in recent years, so has the prevalence of compulsive online sexual behavior. This second edition is updated with the latest information, equipping readers with specific strategies for recognizing and changing compulsive sexual behaviors.

Cruise Control: Understanding Sex Addiction in Gay Men
by Robert Weiss.

Avoiding political and moral arguments, this book focuses on the clinical approach, asking the question, "Is your sexual behavior causing problems in other areas of your life?" Cruise Control leads men to a better understanding of the difference between sexual compulsion and non-addictive sexual behavior within the gay experience, and it explains what resources are available for recovery.

The Porn Trap: The Essential Guide To Overcoming Problems Caused By Pornography
By Wendy Maltz and Larry Maltz

In this recovery guide, sex and relationship therapists Wendy and Larry Maltz shed new light on the compelling nature and destructive power of today's instantly available pornography. Weaving together real-life stories with exercises, checklists, and expert advice, this resource provides a comprehensive program for understanding and healing porn addiction and other serious consequences of porn use.

Don't Call It Love: Recovery from Sexual Addiction
by Patrick Carnes, Ph.D.

Based on the candid testimony of more than one thousand recovering sexual addicts in the first major scientific study of the disorder. This volume includes not only the findings of Dr. Carne's research with recovering addicts but also advice from the addicts and their partners as they work to overcome their compulsive behavior.

Untangling the Web
by Jennifer Schneider and Robert Weiss.

With personal stories from addicts and their significant others, this updated resource offers realistic healing strategies for anyone experiencing the devastating impact of Internet pornography and sex addiction on intimacy, relationships, career, health, and self-respect.

Confronting Pornography: A Guide to Prevention and Recovery for Individuals, Loved Ones, and Leaders
By Mark D. Chamberlain

A collection of articles from professional counselors, leaders, and individuals who have dealt with pornography problems personally, this useful book is an invaluable resource. It offers understanding, powerful tools based in gospel principles, and, most of all, hope.

Acknowledgements

First and foremost I want to thank my clients who made this book possible. Their work and dedication to their process flushed out the experiences in Letters.

In so many ways I was supported to write and make this book a reality. H.P. gets highest billing along with David Sawyer, Brenna Hopkins, Chris Thatcher, Sonya Shannon and Valerie Lorig. In addition, there were dozens of people who through this process have said kind and encouraging words that helped perhaps more than you know.

My editor, Marianne Harkin, was the best mid-wife I could imagine. My Certified Sex Addiction community helped continuously, especially Michael Barta and Cindy Power. My teachers Ken Adams, Stephanie Carnes, Patrick Carnes and Rob Weiss have created a tour de force for research and education for sex addiction for which I am grateful. I believe they are missioned to help and heal: they follow that directive with integrity and grace.

If you ask a writer how they wrote their book, usually there is a team involved. My writing team consists of other writers, naturally. Some of them I want to mention by name. Thank you Belle Schmidt and Barbara Hoffman, who read my work for years, and especially during the dark days. Thank you to Susan Piver who is an inspiration for creativity, dedication and discipline. However, specifically for this book, a dear friend gave me a journal after my own experience of Discovery, for which I am ever grateful.

Last, but not least, I want to thank my family, specifically Kerstin, Byron, Tyler, Lyndel, Irene, Ted A and Ted B, Edward L. Benno, and all the horses. You have been there for me through the best and worst of times.

About the Author

Wendy Conquest, MA, LPC, CSAT-S is a national speaker, teacher, writer, and therapist. She has developed multiple programs dealing with drug, alcohol, and sex addiction in addition to treating partners of sex addicts. Ms. Conquest has served as director, clinical director, and clinical supervisor for various treatment facilities along the front range of Colorado.

Her experience covers working with children, step-families, high conflict divorce, sexual abuse, couples, and families, as well as treating sex addicts and partners of sex addicts. She has extensive training and experience working with trauma, and employs multiple modalities in her work, including EMDR, BrainSpotting, Integrative Body Psychotherapy (IBP), and equine assisted psychotherapy.

Ms. Conquest is a Certified Sex Addiction Therapist as well as a supervisor for those in training.

Made in the USA
Las Vegas, NV
17 November 2024

12023287R00104